St. Paul Chiropractor Reveals:
48 Self Strategies to Stop and Prevent Back Pain

Dr. Joel Fugleberg

First Printing, 2010

ISBN 1456331892

Printed in the United States of America

About The Author

Dr. Joel Fugleberg is a St. Paul area chiropractor at Lifestyle Chiropractic in Mendota Heights.

Dr. Fugleberg is a member of both the Minnesota Chiropractic Association and the American Chiropractic Association. He has helped hundreds of people get well with chiropractic and natural health strategies and loves sharing information that will benefit others on this path.

In his spare time, Dr. Fugleberg most enjoys spending time with his family and staying active. Currently, he has two kids under the age of 3 that help him accomplish both of those goals!

Contact Dr. Fugleberg by visiting his website at:

www.LifestyleChiroCenter.com

DISCLAIMER:

The information in this publication is not intended or implied to be a substitute for professional medical advice, diagnosis or treatment. All content, including text, graphics, images and information, contained on or available through this publication is for general information purposes only. If other expert assistance is required, personal consultation with a medical or other healthcare professional or the services of a competent healthcare professional should be sought.

Stop Screen Strain

A very common source of pain for many in today's society is computer usage. Straining to focus on your monitor may not be painful for several minutes or even hours, but compound that by 8 hours a day, 5 days a week, 52

weeks in a year and you quickly log over 2000 hours of muscle strain and fatigue! Turn your monitor so it is directly in front of you so you don't have to turn to look at it. Raise it to eye level so you can gaze comfortably at the screen without your chin nodding downward.

Stop Smoking

S moking is obviously not a healthy habit. But when it comes to pain and recovery from pain there may be nothing worse. Smoking constricts blood vessels and prevents good circulation to potentially damaged

Back Pain

tissues. Smoking causes a buildup of toxic substances that prolong the healing process and prevent your body from responding quickly.

Look Up When You Pick Up

This simple mantra repeated prior to lifting will prevent tons of back pain! Rather than focusing on the object you are picking up, put your focus straight in front of you. Extend your head up and back. By

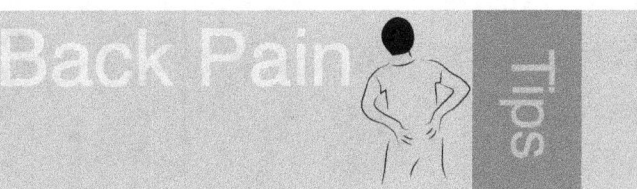

looking up, you ensure good posture, engage the proper muscles and prevent potential injury.

Bounce On A Ball

You've seen the core exercise balls. Sometimes they're called Swiss balls. Toss the office chair and sit on this instead. Doing so activates your core musculature and reduces fatigue. It also promotes circulation since you will not be sitting still. The

discs in your spine get their nutrients from movement so this helps prevent disc degeneration. Many workplaces and even schools are utilizing Swiss balls for better focus and lower risk of injury. Don't want to be "that guy" in the office? Try a Back Vitalizer™ instead.

Position Your Posterior In Your Car

The primary complaint of many patients with back pain is that they can't travel, even short distances without pain. Sadly, car companies have yet to develop a car seat that promotes proper posture in 100% of the public. After all, we're all different! So the responsibility is yours. Place your seat back at such an

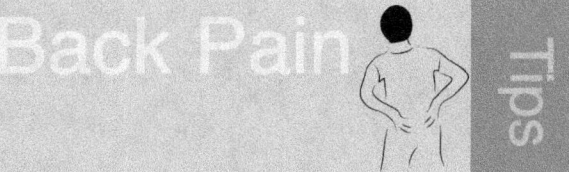

Back Pain Tips

angle that your head can rest comfortably against your head rest. Move your seat forward so your hands rest comfortably against your steering wheel with a slight bend in your elbows. Maintain the curve in your lower back with a lumbar support cushion.

5

Break In Your Bed

The best solution is a custom mattress that allows custom firmness. This is especially important if your spouse requires a different level of firmness (as is the case for the majority of couples). A third of our life is spent sleeping so why not be

Back Pain

Tips

comfortable during this time? Most spring mattresses have a life of less than 5 years so a custom mattress is the way to go. Select Comfort™ and iSleep™ are two of the best brands currently available. Both offer trial periods to test their product to see if it is right for you.

Wear Shoes With Support

T ypically the best shoes are athletic shoes. They tend to conform to our feet better and also provide support for foot structure. Find a pair that fit

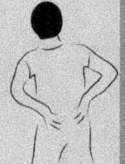

Back Pain Tips

properly and buy several pairs. Then if that particular style is discontinued you won't be left high and dry having to research a new pair. This applies to work boots, dress shoes, and other footwear. Buy for support first. Ordering a pair of custom-fit orthotics for your shoes is even better. Trust me, your feet and back will thank-you.

Ditch The High Heels

B efore you stab me with a stiletto, hear me out. Most people buy for fashion first and sacrifice comfort. It's not uncommon to see women prancing around in high-heeled shoes

Back Pain

wincing in pain! Aside from risk of turning an ankle or falling, high heels can cause a host of problems: Morton's neuroma, metatarsalgia, spondylolisthesis, and many other painful conditions. If you don't know what those are, that's good. Don't wear high heels and maybe you never will!

8

Use Proper Form
When Pumping Iron

C ould there be any more important time for good posture than when lifting weights? If you are training your muscles in the gym don't fail to use proper posture. Failing to do so turns a healthy habit into a

Back Pain

Tips

poor one! Engage your core. Use support belts when necessary. Lifting weights properly strengthens the body and helps promote balance. A balanced body prevents potential injury. But use proper posture.

9

Strengthen Your Core

Your routine of morning crunches is not enough to have a strong core. Your abdominals are always activated when you perform any movement. The transverses abominus (TA) is a corset-like muscle that wraps your midsection. To strengthen this

 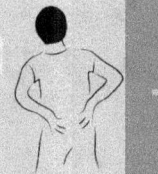

muscle, try the plank position. Lie flat on your stomach on the floor or a yoga mat. Raise your body so that your upper body is supported on your elbows by your forearms and your lower body on your toes. You should feel pressure around your midsection. Your body should be straight and resemble a plank.

Go Shopping

No, I don't mean to spend a ton of money at the mall. While that may be cathartic, there is a more practical aspect at play here. Light exercise and stretching of your legs may be necessary to reduce your healing time. If you are in a lot of pain,

Back Pain

Tips

exercise may not be possible. Go to the store, grab a shopping cart and take laps around the aisles like you are intent on finding an item. This may be just the ticket to spurring on faster healing and stretching your legs with very little resistance.

Stretch Your Piriformis

You've undoubtedly heard of piriformis syndrome. This painful condition is caused from tightening of the piriformis muscle at the hip joint and buttocks. Too much tension here pinches the sciatic nerve causing

pain. Stretch the piriformis by sitting with the affected leg crossed like a figure-four on your opposite leg. Interlock your fingers around your knee and pull your knee up and across your body until you feel a nice stretch in your buttock and hip muscle. Hold 20-30 seconds.

Stop Stomach
Sleeping

Imagine turning your head as far to the left as you can and holding it in that position for 8 hours. Ouch! The muscles of your neck would shorten or stretch. Fatigue would set in and

Back Pain

Tips

there could be cramping. And yet, this is what you are doing every night when you sleep on your stomach. Invest in a good orthopedic pillow that helps you sleep comfortably on your back or side. You'll sleep better and have less pain.

Support Your Hips
While You Sleep

D ue to large muscle groups along your legs and hips, tension can develop while lying on your side. If you are a side sleeper and experience discomfort sleeping, try this. Place a small throw pillow between your

Back Pain

Tips

knees. This serves to relieve some pressure on your hips and lower back.

Firm Up Your Foundation

Do you stand long periods?
Do you run or walk?
Consider some support for
the arches of your feet. Most
orthotics or supports only address
the inside arch, but your feet have

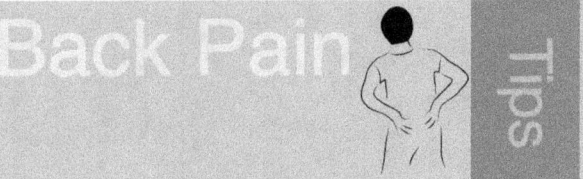

Back Pain Tips

3 arches. Get orthotics custom fit
for your feet to provide stability for
the rest of your body.

Stand On Softer Surfaces

A very common aggravation for workers is the concrete or tiled floor they stand on. Even standing on kitchen floors can cause pain! If standing for long periods gives you a backache, consider an anti-fatigue floor mat

Back Pain Tips

to stand on. These mats provide a cushion for you to stand on and greatly reduce strain on your postural muscles.

Do the "D"

Vitamin D has been shown to be effective at aiding a whole host of things. One of these things is the prevention of back pain. Are your levels adequate? We naturally produce vitamin D

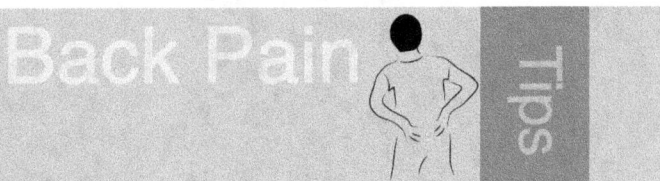
Back Pain Tips

when our skin is exposed to sunlight. A supplement can be a good idea especially in the winter months.

17

Take Some Fish Oil

Fish oil is a source of Omega 3 fat which is essential for our bodies. We typically don't get enough of this in our diet so supplementing this is a must for most. This helps reduce

Back Pain

Tips

inflammation and pain, among many other things. Be careful. Not all fish oil is the same. Look for a high-quality fish oil that has been certified as free of impurities!

Don't Degenerate

Your spinal discs are filled with fluid. This is held in place by special molecules. Chondroitin sulfate, glucosamine, and hyaluronic acid are some of the main ones. If these degenerate you may experience pain and

Back Pain

Tips

dysfunction. Age, time, and misalignment of your spinal bones are some of the factors that may cause degenerative discs. Delay the degeneration and promote regeneration with a chondroitin or glucosamine supplement.

When To Ice

The rule of thumb is to use ice for the first 72 hours after an injury. You can use ice after that too, but it is most useful to help halt early inflammation. Don't overdo it. You should only ice for 15-20 minutes at a time.

Back Pain

Tips

Use an ice pack, a bag of ice, or even a bag of frozen vegetables to apply the ice therapy. Just cover your skin with a light towel before applying the ice pack.

When To Heat

Heat can often be used to reduce muscle spasm. However, it is more useful for chronic pain than acute. It should generally not be used in the first 72 hours following an injury. After that it is useful for relaxing

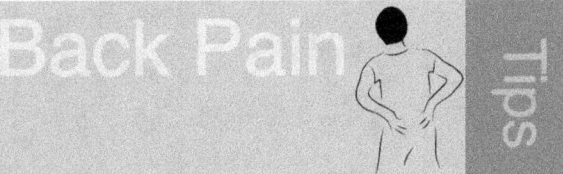

Back Pain Tips

tight muscles and drawing blood flow and more circulation into the muscle tissue. It often feels good and soothes achy muscles.

Don't Dehydrate

K eep the discs in your back
healthy by staying hydrated.
A good rule of thumb is to
drink half your body weight in
ounces of water. For example, a
150 lb person should aim to drink

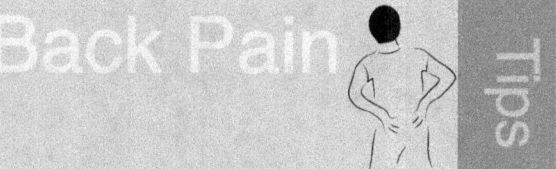

Back Pain Tips

at least 75 ounces of water per
day.

Shun The Spirits

Drinking certain fluids will actually cause dehydration in your body. Coffee, tea and alcohol can act as diuretics in your body leaving you dehydrated

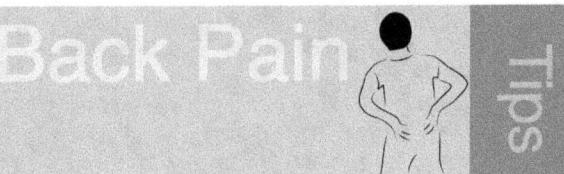

by the end of your day. Dehydration can make you more sensitive to pain signals in your body.

Fast Food

A side from clogging your arteries, fried foods tend to create an imbalance between

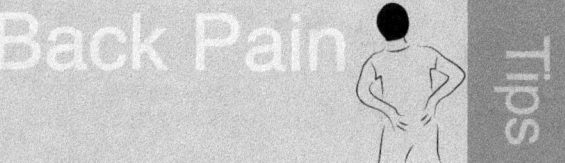

Back Pain

Tips

omega 6 and omega 3 fats in our body. This promotes inflammation. Avoid fried foods and you will feel less pain!

Where's The Fiber?

If you've ever been constipated you know how uncomfortable that can be. You may have flank pain or a back ache.

Back Pain 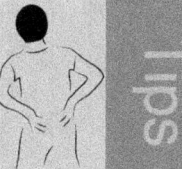 Tips

Sometimes this discomfort can be referred pain from distention in your digestive tract. Eat healthy fiber daily to prevent this.

Spinal Hygiene

Whe know we need to floss and brush daily if we want to have healthy teeth. What do we do to maintain a healthy spine? Moving your spine

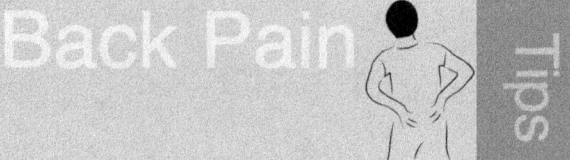

Back Pain Tips

through its full range of motion daily is the first step to a healthy spine and preventing pain.

Maintain Your Spine

Do you only get your oil changed when your engine sputters and smokes? Do you only work out when you

Back Pain

Tips

become overweight? Do you only see your dentist when you get a cavity? Of course not! Then don't only go to your chiropractor when you have back pain. Go regularly to maintain your spine and prevent painful flare-ups.

Don't Be A Weekend Warrior

Just because you could play tackle football without pads as a pre-teen doesn't mean

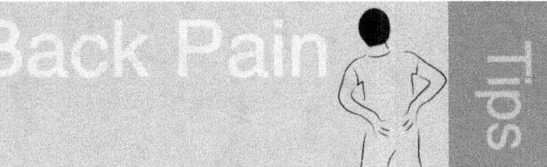

Back Pain

Tips

you should try it as an adult! Many injuries occur by jumping into an activity to soon. Work up to more strenuous activity slowly and avoid weekend warrior pain.

Balance Your Beach Body

T oo many lifters overdevelop their "beach muscles" while neglecting complementary

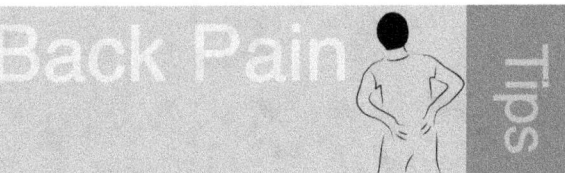
Back Pain Tips

muscle groups. You know the look-huge pectorals and rounded shoulders. This abnormal posture may seem to look good on the beach or in the mirror but is imbalanced and sets the body up for pain and dysfunction.

Stretch At Your Desk

Your hip flexors will shorten and pull your lower back forward if you sit for long periods of time. Stand regularly and stretch your hip flexors at the

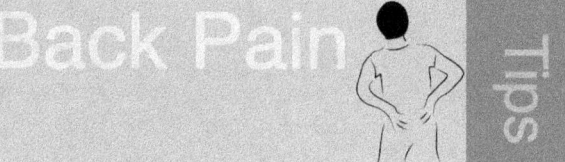

Back Pain Tips

front of your hip. Do this by straightening your leg and leaning forward. This will reduce tension on your lower back.

Lighten Up

Obviously, being overweight is unhealthy for a lot of reasons. Excess weight places stress on the joints and discs of your spine and promotes

poor posture. It also promotes many inflammatory processes that can occur in your body. Maintaining a healthy weight helps correct poor posture and will reduce strain throughout your body.

31

Brace Your Back

In an ideal world your core strength is adequate to protect your back from injury when lifting. In the world we live in, that may not be the case! Protect your

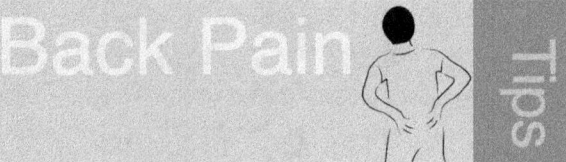

Back Pain

Tips

back using a corset-like brace around your midsection. This locks your core and assists you when lifting heavier objects.

Avoid Inversion

While some people swear by their inversion table or hanging boots, these are not generally recommended. When you hang upside down you are

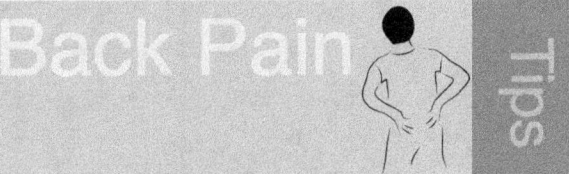

Back Pain Tips

putting an abnormal amount of strain on your back muscles. Your body weight instantly becomes the traction force. This sudden stretch can lead to spasm in your back muscles. Not to mention the potential danger of your boots disconnecting and you falling on your head!

Having Kids Is A Balancing Act

Switch sides when carrying your toddler. Even a small baby can become a

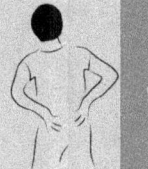

significant physical stress when carried on the same hip. Shift your child to the other hip and displace at least some of the tension that comes with young children!

34

Practice Good Purse Posture

Posture assessment in many women reveal a high shoulder on one side when compared

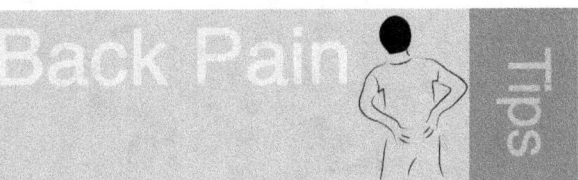

to the other. This can be due to carrying a heavy purse primarily on that side. The muscles compensate and become tense. Consequently the overall posture is compromised and becomes imbalanced. Switch shoulders and minimize the weight of your handbag!

Don't Slump And Cycle

R iding a Harley may be cool but it's not the best practice for the health of your spine.

Back Pain

Tips

The sloped seats on most cycles cause a slouched posture and place stress on the discs of the spine.

Bend At The Knees

When you pick up an object, take care to notice where you are bending. Most

often the bulk of the bend is in your back. Bend at your knees, keeping your back straight if possible. Not only will you prevent pain and injury, you'll be able to lift more!

Stop Twisting

T ry to avoid using twisting motions especially when lifting heavy objects but even

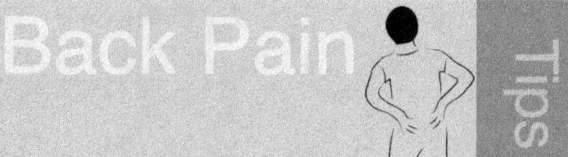

Back Pain

Tips

when doing simple tasks such as house cleaning. Your spine is at its weakest when you are bent over and twisted so avoid putting your spine in a compromised position.

Don't "Crack"

One of the worst things to do is to try to "crack" your own back. Bending over a chair or counter or even resorting to someone walking on your back can

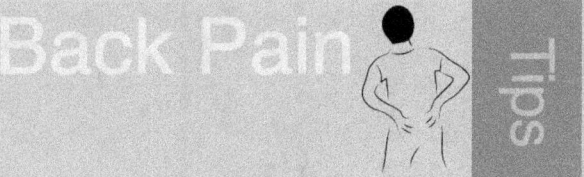

Back Pain

Tips

put your spine out of alignment and cause further pain.

Pick the Right Shovel

If you're fortunate to live somewhere with high snow banks in the winter, be sure to choose the correct type of snow shovel. Using incorrect body mechanics can cause strain and pain and the proper shovel will aid

 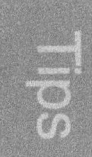

good posture while you shovel. A curved ergonomic handle is best to allow minimal bending as you lift the snow while keeping the blade on the ground. Most hardware stores will have this option. Or better yet, hire the neighbor kid to shovel!

Stretch Slowly

You have heard of the importance of stretching. But equally, if not more important is the importance of proper stretching. Ease into the stretch. Allow time for your muscle fibers to slowly elongate. Allow the blood to circulate as you lean into your

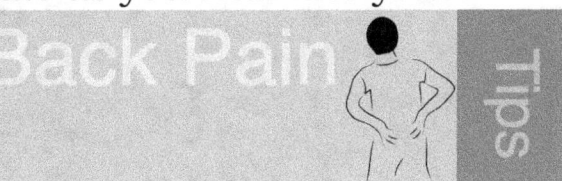

Back Pain Tips

stretch. Above all-don't bounce!

Whip Out Your Wallet

N o, I don't mean it's going to be expensive to prevent pain. But pulling your wallet out of your pocket is a key secret. Simply remove your wallet from your back pocket before sitting. Period. Thick wallet or thin, sitting

Back Pain

on it puts uneven pressure on your pelvis and can lead to misalignment and pain.

Unpack The Backpack

Most kids carry backpacks that are way too heavy for their frame. The American Chiropractic Association recommends that the bag your

Back Pain

Tips

child carries should be loaded as a percentage of their body weight. It should weigh no more than 5-10% of their body weight.

Lift In Stages

This can be a key strategy for a variety of tasks. Lifting heavy objects can be made easier if the lift is broken up into several smaller lifts. This applies to lifting luggage. When you're traveling you may not be thinking about

Back Pain

Tips

good biomechanics when hurrying to stuff your suitcase into the overhead compartment. But try this. Lift the luggage to the top of the seat first, then change your position and lift to the overhead compartment.

44

Get A Massage

If you've ever had a good massage, I probably don't need to convince you how good it feels. Massage warms up and relaxes your muscles. It stimulates your body's sensory nerves and helps decrease pain signals by releasing your body's

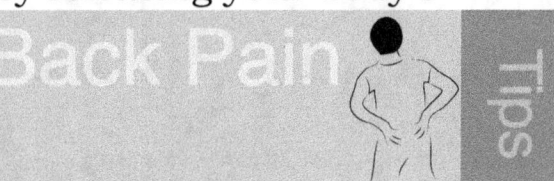

Back Pain Tips

endorphins – your natural pain-killers. It will even enhance your immunity by stimulating lymph flow – part of your natural defense system.

Move!

Long hours at the computer, sitting in front of the television, or taking a road trip are recipes for pain. Motion is life. Take frequent breaks. Do not remain sedentary. Get up and move and you will naturally feel less pain.

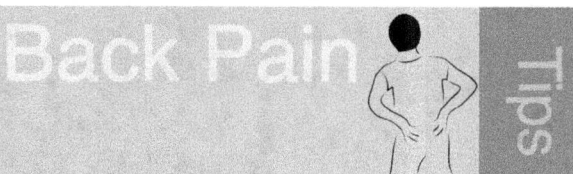

Back Pain Tips

Push, Don't Pull

Generally, it is better to try and push heavier objects than to try and pull them. This engages the large muscles of your legs and hips rather than focusing the strain on your lower back. Try this the next time you move your couch, dresser or piano.

Back Pain Tips

Keep It Close

When lifting or carrying an object, try to carry it close to the trunk of your body. The closer it is to your body, the less strain you will feel. Keep objects tight to your torso and you will have less chance of injury.

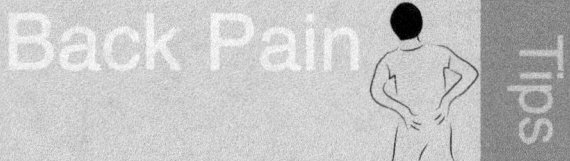

Back Pain

Tips

www.ingramcontent.com/pod-product-compliance
Lightning Source LLC
Chambersburg PA
CBHW071254280526
45788CB00004B/1717